Animal Science Reviews

Vol. 1

Animal Science Reviews

Vol. 1

SSPH

403, Express Tower, Commercial Complex
Azadpur, Delhi-110033 (India)
Phone : 011-27672852, Fax : 91-11-27672046
E-mail :info@satishserial.com, hkjain1975@yahoo.com
Website : www.satishserial.com

Published by :

SATISH SERIAL PUBLISHING HOUSE
403, Express Tower, Commercial Complex, Azadpur,
Delhi-110033 (INDIA)
Phone : 011-27672852 Fax : 91-11-27672046
E-mail : info@satishserial.com, hkjain1975@yahoo.com

ISBN 978-93-81226-35-3

Typeset at: Harminder Singh Kharb *for* Laxmi Art Creation
Printed at: Salasar Imaging Systems, Delhi-110035

Preface

We are very much happy to offer you the first volume of Animal Science Reviews Hopefully, Now onwards the animal science reviews will be published regularly. Hope this review will be helpful to serve the scientific community with latest and advanced information regarding the advancement of animal science research in India and abroad. The animal science reviews is published with its aim to update scientific news & current issues and make aware to the scientific community with the latest advancement. Our mandate is to collect the new and latest information from scientific personnel for published it to cater the needs of research reviews to the scientific fraternity including students working in animal science. It is decided that the very latest information will be published in animal science reviews every year. We believe that the scientific personnel will always help us by contributing their writings, so that we will be able to publish it in a proper manner, proper time and able to cover every aspect in animal science. We can assure you with your valuable help and cooperation that it will be a very good publication and would be a very useful for researchers, teachers and students. We invite your valuable comments and suggestions for its further improvements in future volumes. We also request the scientist, teachers, students and entrepreneurs to submit articles and news for publication for future volumes. At the end I extent our heartfelt thanks to the contributors for contributing good articles for publishing this book and the publisher M/s. Satish Serial Publishing House, Delhi for helping me by publishing the reviews in a befitting manner. I also extend my sincere thanks to editorial board for helping me to publish it in a proper shape.

S.K. Saha
Chief Editor

Contents

Contents

Chapter 1

Feeding of Dairy Animals : Problems and Remedies

N. K. S. GOWDA AND K. T. SAMPATH
National Institute of Animal Nutrition and Physiology
Adugodi, Bangalore- 560 030

Dairying is a major economical activity that provides employment and economic opportunities to many. Amongst the many factors influencing profitable dairying, feeding accounts for about 60-70% of the total input and hence any improvement in feeding aspect of dairy cattle will have greater impact on the productivity.

Feed resources

As crop resides continue to be the major source of roughage for livestock, there is a need to improve their nutritive value both in terms of their intake and digestion. Enriching the crop residues with ammoniation has shown promising benefits but has been little adopted at field level. Supplementation in the form of urea, molasses and minerals would help in improving the rumen fermentation and microbial activity, thereby improving feed utilization, concept of complete feeds or total mixed ration allow incorporation of crop residues and unconventional feds along with concentrate ingredients in a uniform mixture of mash or pellet by employing grinding, mixing and extruding process. Feeding complete feeds makes rumen environment more stable with reduced energy losses and stabilize the acetate to propionate ratio. Poor quality roughage utilization can be improved through complete fees because of the readily available nitrogen and energy. Meeting the protein requirement though conventional oil cake has become expensive. Presence of certain anti-nutritional factors in some unconventional protein – rich feeds has limited their safe inclusion in cattle diets. Chemical treatment of neem seed cake, mustrard cake, karanj cake, castor seed cake etc. has shown promising result in utilizing such material as cattle feed. Such technologies need to be upscaled at industrial level for their regular usage in diary concentrate mixture. Feeding of green fodder is very important for economizing the dairy production. At least 30-40 % of the dry matter requirement should be met through feeding good quality green fodder. Supplementation of legume fodders like Lucerne or berseem to straw based diets, improves fiber digestibility.

Protein and Energy

High yielding dairy animals require better quality protein in their diet in terms of essential amino acids, particularly lysine and methionine, which are deficient in rumen microbial protein. During early lactation, dry matter intake is low due to pregnancy and parturition stress. For sustaining high milk yield, the diet has to be adequate in both available energy and protein. Rumen microbial protein is to be complemented and/ or supplemented to provide adequate amino acids to maximize milk production and milk protein content. Based on the qualification of methionine and lysine as limiting amino acids for milk protein synthesis, diets can be evaluated based on available amino acids. Rumen microbes too have a requirement for protein and their efficiency of protein synthesis can be improved by feeding rumen degradable protein, but not to exceed their requirement. For high producing diary cattle, even when rumen microbial protein output is maximized, still not enough protein enteres small intestine to realize potential milk production. Common protein sources with higher undegradable protein content include animal proteins, com gluten meal, cotton seed meal and copra meal and each selecting protein ingredients for ration formulation. Bypass protein fractions of silkworm pupae, safflower cake and copra cake provide high amount of lysine, while the bypass protein fractions of silkworm pupae, maize gluten meal provide more amount of methiomine. Lysine and methionine are the primary limiting amino acids for diary cows. Supplementing individual amino acid/amino acid analogue to diary cattle has been proved to be beneficial. Incorporation of amino acids prior to parturition stimulates dry matter intake, which contribute significantly to increase in milk production.

The dietary energy requirement of high yielders can not be easily met with cereal grains and oil cakes, particularly during peak lactation. Increasing the dry matter intake is the simplest method to meet higher energy requirement but practically difficult. The hormonal changes associated with parturition stress negatively affect the cow's appetite and the rumen microbial population, which had become adapted to the gestation ration must adapt to the lactation ration. Lower feed intake during early lactation causes weight loss and thus negative energy balance. Feeding more concentrate in the form of cereal grain to balance the energy deficit may also result in undesirable incidences like ruminal acidosis, reduced acetic: propionic acid ratio and low milk fat content. Therefore incorporation with the balance through good quality green fodder.

Fats as high energy density nutrients can also be supplemented to prevent body weight loss. However the rumen is very sensitive to the high level of fat in his diet as physical coating of the fiber limits its digestion. The calcium salts of fatty acids are known as calcium soaps and remain intact in a neutral pH of rumen (6.9-7.1), but dissociate in acid medium of abomasums to calcium and fatty acids. These fatty acids are absorbed efficiently in the intestine. Both saturated fat products and calcium soap are effective in bypassing the rumen and delivering a concentrated source of energy at small intestine.

Minerals

Majority of the reproduction related problems like repeat breeding and anoestrus in dairy cattle have been implicated due to the deficiency and / or imbalance of mineral, particularly trace minerals like Cu, Zn, Mn, and Co. The impairment of reproductive function resulting from these mineral deficiencies are believed to be associated with enzymatic dysfunction. Feeding system where straws and stovers are the major roughages, the bioavailability of certain minerals is likely to below. Elements like selenium, is understood to be essential in preventing disorders like retention of placenta, metritis and mastitis in diary cattle, besides helping to improve the immune function.

High pressure on soil due to modern agricultural practices like potass/ phosphatic fertilizer application results in limited absorption of some minerals from soil to plant/ fodder. Cost-effective practical method of mineral supplementation to the existing traditional feeding system are required to strengthen and sustain the animal productivity. Mineral mixtures are to be formulated keeping in view of their quality and bioavailability. Organic minerals/ chelated mineral ate better bioavailabe than their inorganic salts. Commercially zinc-methionine, copper-caseinate, iron-caseinate, magnese-methionine, copper-lysine complexes are bing produced. Increased milk production and decreased somatic cell count have been observed in lactation cows fed chelated minerals. When dietary molybdenum and sulfur are high in the diet, providing copper in organic form would be more beneficial. Supplementing mineral in the form of area specific mineral mixture is an easy solution for overcoming the mineral deficiency in the diary cattle.

Feed management

A sound late pregnancy – feeding program is a key to improved lactation to loose body weight, which will increase the risk of fatty live syndrome. Niacin can be fed at 4-6 gram per day to maintain dry matter intake and to minimize the risk of ketosis. High quality lush hay/fodder feeding would stimulate appetite and rumen function. The early dry cow ration is to be formulated for higher digestible fiber with medium energy density, while the late gestation ration should contain higher energy density with less fibre. Environmental stresses and drastic dietary changes should be minimized during the transition period from late gestation to lactation.

❑❑❑

Chapter 2

Welfare of Laminitis in Horses

S.DEY[1] AND S.K. SAHA[2]
1 Principal Scientist, Division of Medicine
2 Senior Scientist Division of Animal Nutrition
Indian Veterinary research Institute Izatnagar, Bareilly - 243122

Laminitis is a common problem of horses due to inflammation of the sensitive laminae of the hoof and clinically characterized by excruciating pain, pounding digital pulse and lameness.

Though, the cause of laminitis is unknown, several factors like excessive ingestion of grain, mechanical concussion, toxaemia, severe systemic infections, stress and ingestion of lush grass & toxic plants are incriminated as causative factors for laminitis in equine. Obesity, diet and systemic illness increase the individual risk. Similarly, ill managemental practice like excessive work on hard surface is also responsible for development of such condition.

Clinical signs

- Pounding digital pulse felt in the palmer digital artery.

- Pain and lameness.
- Shifting weight between the feet.
- Standing on heals to relieve pressure on feet.
- Reluctant to lift feet and move.
- Frequent lying down.

The condition may turn into chronic form if proper treatment and management are not followed up. If chronic form of laminitis occurs neither the animal died nor it recover and remained as a permanent cripple till death. The signs of chronic laminitis are:

- Intermittent lameness and severe pain.
- Rotation of Pedal bone.
- Diverging growth of the hoof wall with visible structural deformity.
- Separation of wall from sensitive laminae.
- Dropping of sole.
- Decubiturs ulcer if there is prolongs recumbency.

Diagnosis

Laminitis can be diagnosed by close observation of clinical symptoms and physical examination of the patient. *It is easy to diagnose laminitis but it is difficult to ascertain the cause of laminitis.*

Treatment and Control

Attempt should be made to locate and remove the cause of laminitis first. After that the following measures should be followed for therapeutic management of laminitis

1. Minimize movement of the animals.
2. *Provide foot Frog rest.* (Roller Bar Shoe maybe used in such condition).
3. Provide relief of Pain.
   - Any of the following drugs can be used Phenylbutazone @ 2.2-4.4 mg/kg, intravenously twice daily till disappeared of pain.

   OR

   - Flunixin meglumine @ 1.1 mg/kg, intramuscularly or intravenously twice daily for 4-5 days/disappears of pain.

   OR

   - Ketophen @ 2.2 mg/kg, intramuscularly twice daily for 4-5 days or till disappearance of pain.

   OR

   - Dimethyl sulfoxide @ 1 gm/kg, intravenously as a 10% solution in normal saline solution can be given in acute laminitis once daily for 6-7 days. Besides its anti inflammatory action it can also remove free radical mediated damages.
4. *Create vasodilatation of the blood vessels of the foot.*

Any of the following drugs can be used.

- Acetylpromazine @ 0.01-0.05 mg/kg, intramuscularly, thrice daily for 4-5 days.
- Isoxuprine @ 1.0 -1.5 mg/kg, orally twice daily for 3-4 days.
- Glyceryl trinitrate (15-30 mg/ artery daily) may be used locally over the palmar digital arteries of the affected limbs to increase blood flow.

5. *Prevention of micro thrombi formation.*

- Aspirin @ 10 mg/kg, orally after every 2 days for 2-3 occasions.
- Heparin @ 40-80 IU/kg, intravenously, thrice daily for 3-4 days.

6. *Promotion of healing*

- Methionine @ 10gm daily for 3 days followed by 5 gm daily for 10 days can be given to both acute and chronic laminitis. It helps in formation of chondrotin complex of collagen and promotes healing.

7. *Improvement of managemental conditions.*

- Mechanical support to frog/sole by use of roller bar shoe.
- Cold water foots both to relief acute pain.

Do's	**Don'ts**
Provide fibre intake >1% of body weight.	Restrict intake of large Quantity of lush grass (which contain water soluble Fructan)
Feed stemmy hay	Never starve or over fed with grain.
Feed Soya oil (small quantity along with feed).	Do not feed to much starchy cereal meal.
Always use feed supplement such as vitamin, A, C & E.	Do not allow horses to stand >12 hr. during Journey.
Provide flavinoid rice feed to improve circulation	Do not use corticosteroid, xylazine enrofloxacin and detomidine in horse with laminitis.
Provide mild exercise to the ailing animal	Do no take excess work on hard surface.

Chapter 3

Nutrition and Feeding of Mithun in NEH Region of India

K.C. DAS, B. PRAKASH, K.K. BARUAH* & C. RAJKHOWA
* C.V Sc, AAU, Khanapara, Guwahati, Assam
NRC on Mithun, Jharnapani, Medziphema, Nagaland

Introduction

North-Eastern Hilly region of India is endowed with diverse plant and animal resources. Vast area of NE region is covered with forest and many species of plants and animals are seen in this region. Mithun (*Bos frontalis*), is an important animal of North-Eastern hilly region of India. Mithun is considered to be the domesticated form of wild gaur (*Bos gaurus*) and it is an extremely efficient grazer on steep hilly slopes compared to other animals. This unique bovine species is believed to be domesticated more than 8000 years ago and is mainly available in the four North-Eastern hilly states of India i.e. Arunachal Pradesh, Nagaland, Mizoram and Manipur. Besides, mithun is also available in Jammu and Kashmir. According to the 2003 livestock census, total mthun population in India is 0.28 million out of which 1,92,000 animals are available in Arunachal Pradesh followed by 40,000 in Nagaland, 24,000 in Jammu and Kashmir, 20,000 in Manipur and 2,000 in Mizoram. This region is covered with forest and tree leaves/shrubs are available in plenty for feeding of mithun. Tree leaves are cheap source of nutrients like protein, vitamins and minerals. But many tree leaves contain various levels of antinutritional factors that have an affinity for carbohydrate, amino acids and minerals rendering them unavailable for rumen microflora and host animal (Makkar, 2003). However proper scientific knowledge of tree leaves and feeding of tree leaves containing good nutritional composition is the correct steps for best utilization of these natural resources.

Tree leaves as cheap source of nutrients

The North East India is covered with forests. The tree foliages are available in plenty. Tree forages not only provide a cheap source of nitrogen, energy and micronutrients but also have many other advantages like their laxative influence on the alimentary system, low degradability of nitrogen in the rumen, and above all the scope of adding variety to the diet. Tree foliage is natural source of bypass protein in the diet of ruminants. They contain certain endogenous secondary plant compounds to bind with protein and protect them from microbial attack. The condensed tannin present in tree leaves is used as organic protectant of proteins. When condensed tannin containing herbage is masticated, condensed tannin protein complexes are formed, these are stable over the pH range of 3.5-7 but dissociate in the abomasums and anterior duodenum. This protects the protein from microbial hydrolysis and deamination in the rumen and increases the proportion of dietary amino acids available for postruminal absorption, since the tannin protein complex is assumed to dissociate at low pH of abomasums. Condensed tannins are claimed to have the potential to modify rumen fermentation. However higher levels of condensed tannins are reported to negatively affect rumen fermentation. Many of the tree leaves and shrubs available in NE region for feeding of mthun were identified and analysed for chemical composition. The tree leaves and grasses consumed by mithun have been analysed and compared in terms of chemical composition. As per the findings, DM content of the grasses varied between 13.28 and 47.62, ash between 8.60 and 13.80, CP between 50.60 and 12.81, EE between 1.10 and 3.08% and total carbohydrate between 72.92 and 83.43% respectively. The corresponding values for the tree leaves were 20.06 and 47.46, 3.0 and 18.86, 9.83 and 21.00, 1.44 and 6.56 and 61.10 and 84.70 percent respectively. Fibre components of the grasses and tree leaves ranged from: NDF, 38.92-76.06 and 37.10-

58.86; ADF, 25.94-47.94 and 17.21-41.64 and hemicellulose from 12.98-34.26 and 5.13-28.98 percent respectively. It was observed that ash and fibre fraction were comparatively higher in grasses than tree leaves where as CP was higher in tree leaves than grasses. About 200 species of tree leaves/shrubs collected from different pockets of NEH region have been analysed and as per findings, the tree leaves/shrubs like *Trema orientalis, Ficus hirta, Ficus hookerii, Lagerstroemia spp, Quercus polystachya, Melia azadiracta, Adenosacme longifoli,* were found to be promising available in this region. As per general findings tree leaves and shrubs contain more protein compared to cultivated fodder.

Effect of tree leaves supplementation on performance of animals

Tree leaves/shrubs feeding are a common practice in hilly states of NE region. This system of feeding is not only practical but also appears to be somewhat scientific. Systematic work has been done on feeding of tree leaves/shrubs which are available in plenty and are also relished by the mithun. *Lagerstroemia speciosa* (Thumero) is one of the important tree foliage having good nutritive value (8 %DCP and 48 %TDN). It is liked by mithun under natural browsing condition. Inclusion of *Lagerstroemia speciosa* as green foliage showed higher daily body weight gain, dry matter (DM) intake and feed conversion ratio in growing mithuns. *Lagerstroemia speciosa* tree leaves can be incorporated successfully up to 30% (on DM basis) for feeding of growing mithuns. Similarly *Ficus hirta* and *Borrena hirticulata* are other important foliages in the NEH region and can be incorporated in the diet of mithun. Cherry leaves (*Pranus cerasoides*) and tophala(*Borrena hirticulata)* leaves are available in Nagaland. Cherry leaves and tophala leaves in 1:1 ratio along with concentrate mixture had better performance in mithun. However, feeding of mixed tree leaves was found to be practical and scientific in stead of using one or two tree leaves. It provides a variety to the diet. Growth rate of animals were found to be satisfactory after feeding mixed tree leaves based ration to growing mithun. The tree leaves consisted of temechiedie (*Ficus hirta*), Pedu (*Debrogesia longifolia*), thenha (Litsea sps) and thumero (Legroestromea spaciosa). So mixed tree leaves based diet can be a good & practical method for feeding of mithun.

Strategies for Feeding of Mithun

Many tree leaves / shrubs in NEH region were found to be rich source of protein. Tao(*Ficus roxburghii)*, Tayir(*Litsea cintreta*), Remter(*Mastersia assamica*),Yare(*Piper peticellosum*), Byake (*Solanum kurzii*), Tatumnalu(*Pilea glaberrima*) of Arunachal Pradesh, Thumero (*Lagerstroemia speciosa*),

Thedie (*Trema orientalis*), Khusia (*Melia azadiracta*), Tophala(*Borrena hirticulata*) Thenha (Litsea sp.), Tambuinei (*Callicarpa vestita*), Medzei (*Spondias pinnata*), Khramhu (Murus spp) of Nagaland, Thangsam (*Chromolena odorata*), Pangbal (*Manihot esculenta*), Thanrawng (*Gmelina arborea*), Phulrua (*Dendrocalamus hamiltonii*), Vankpuithal (*Bides bidernata*), Theibate *(Ficus auriculata*) of Mizoram and Nake (*Callicarpa arborea*), Vaopa (*Bauhinia hookeri*), Shakhikeng (*Solanum* spp), Lhakhai (*Urtica dioica),* Anthudul (*Herpetospermum spp),* Sheijeplhem (*Herpetospermum spp*) of Manipur were found to be rich in crude protein. These tree leaves may be fed to mithun as rich source of protein. When the tannin level and other antinutritional substance in the tree leaves are more these may be supplemented with other tree leaves or straw containing less tannin. Similarly many tree leaves were found to be rich source of energy. The combination of good source of protein and energy prepares a good type of diet for mithun. The tree leaves containing good source of minerals like calcium can not be ignored as it is an important minerals for growth and milk production. The efficacy of the diet is improved if the mixture of tree leaves/shrubs is fed to mithun in stead of one or two. In this situation the tannin and other antinutritional substances are diluted and animal gets good type of diet.

Vegetative propagation of tree foliages

As per observation in the NE region, there is large-scale deforestation and alteration of habitat of animals because of urbanization, shifting cultivation, jungle fire etc. The availability of tree leaves/shrubs is also not uniform throughout the year. In this situation propagation of fodder tree in NEH region like Nagaland, Manipur, Arunachal Pradesh and Mizoram is the best alternative for making available of sufficient quantity of tree leaves for the animals. Though seed is the main method for multiplication of fodder tree species under natural condition, propagation through vegetative means gives an opportunity to shorten the period of multiplication. Raising planting stock by vegetative propagation, especially by stem cuttings is the possible means in the process of fast multiplication. Plant growth hormones like auxins, cytokinins and combination of both have been tried in NRC Mithun, Nagaland for shortening this process.

The propagation study at NRC on Mithun, Nagaland by using higher dosage of auxins (Indole acetic acid IAA @ 250 ppm) on good quality fodder trees revealed encouraging trend with highest survival percentage, increased length and number of sprouts per stem cuttings (Prakash *et al.* 2007).The selected fodder tree species (*Ficus hirta, Ficus roxburghii, Lagerstroemia speciosa,*

Trema orientalis, Ficus hookeri) can grow meaningfully through stem cuttings treated with IAA which can provide better option for multiplication in degraded pasture land of low carrying capacity.

Important fodder trees/grass for Mithun

Basing on the availability, nutrient composition and acceptance of fodder tree by the farmers for feeding the mithun, few different species have been found to have the major contribution for meeting the fodder requirement for this animal in all mithun inhabited states.

1. *Ficus hirta* (Themichedie)

Genus: *Ficus*

Family: *Moraceae*

This tree found mostly in mid altitude areas of Mithun inhabited states and remains green throughout years. Around 3-4 lopping can be obtained a years with an average fodder yield per cuttings is 64-150 kg/tree (fresh basis). This tree is named as Temechiedie and Heshlak in Angami and Konyak dominated areas of Nagaland, respectively. In Arunachal Pradesh it is called as Nyeihi where it also very much popular for feeding the mithun and other livestock.

2. *Trema orientalis* (Thedie)

Genus: *Trema*

Family:Celtidaceae/Ulmaceae

English name of this tree is pigeon wood. Depending on climatic conditions, trees may be evergreen or deciduous. In forests it is a straight, slender tree grows up to 18 m. The trees are generally found in the higher rainfall areas of northeastern states of India. It occurs in a variety of habitats and is usually found in moist soils. The fruit, leaves, bark, stems, twigs and seeds are used as traditional medicine in Nagaland and Mizoram. In Nagaland, Arunachal Pradesh and Mizoram it's called with local name as Thedie, Yal and Belphuar respectively. An average fodder yield is around 45-110 kg/tree (fresh basis) and 2-3 lopping can be obtained a year. It is common belief among the farmers that the feeding of *Trema orientalis* leaves to the animals' results in increase the milk production.

3. *Ficus hookerii* (Khaboo)

Genus: Ficus

Family: Moraceae

This tree found mostly in high altitude areas (above 1000 m asl) of NEH region. The survivability of this tree is very less at low altitude areas (below 500 m asl). This tree bears a broad leaves which provides green fodder throughout year. 3-5 lopping can be obtained in a year and around 65-135 kg/ tree (fresh basis) green foliage can be attained for feeding the mithuns. This tree can be easily propagated by stem cuttings and through seeds as well. This tree can be transplanted all along the border area of agriculture land in hilly area which gives a greater strength to the fencing of agriculture land.

4. *Lagerstroemia spp.* (Thumero)

Family: *Lagerstroemeaceae*

This tree is abundantly available in low to mid altitude areas (300-1500 m asl) and remains green throughout year. This tree gives 4-5 lopping a year with average green foliage yield of 80-154 kg/tree (fresh basis). The wood of this tree is also used for making the agricultural tools. The tree grows very high, about 8-12 m which gives more fodder yield. This tree is very well propagated through seeds. It is difficult to get sprout from the stem cuttings, unless there is the quite optimum condition under the green house.

5. *Quercus polystachya* (Keromite / Kartoos)

Family: *Fagaceae*

Perennial fodder tree grows rapidly in lower and mid altitude areas of the northeastern

Table 1 : Nutrient composition (% on DM basis) of different foliages collected from Nagaland

Name		Composition % DM basis						
Local	Scientific	CP	EE	CF	NFE	NDF	ADF	Ash
Thumero	*Lagerstroemia speciosa*	23.1	2.10	18.1	49.4	33.0	21.0	7.30
Thedie	*Trema orientalis*	17.1	2.31	28.3	45.9	35.1	25.0	6.40
Pre	*Ficus bengalensis*	15.2	1.91	26.7	48.3	37.0	27.9	7.90
Dzapri	*Oroxylum indicum*	19.8	1.90	27.2	44.8	31.9	23.6	6.30
Khusia	*Melia azadiracta*	26.4	2.30	25.3	37.1	25.0	19.4	8.90
Tego	*Bauhinia hookeri*	21.5	2.01	23.4	43.9	29.7	23.6	9.10
Rambeinei	*Ficus elmeri*	11.9	2.81	18.3	58.2	32.0	21.8	8.70
Heratunei	*Ficus dalhousiae*	22.5	2.47	23.1	46.8	31.0	25.1	5.10
Regapa	*Bauhinia variegata*	15.1	2.51	25.3	51.2	36.2	23.0	5.86
Tambuinei	*Callicarpa vestita*	21.6	2.46	19.3	51.5	38.0	28.0	5.10
Ciesi	*Litsea citrada*	12.2	1.8	26.3	52.5	-	-	7.2
Dzuvo	*Alternanthe ra sesiles*	19.1	2.1	14.6	55.7	-	-	8.5
Tophala	*Borrena hirticulata*	16.0	1.9	22.3	50.7	-	-	9.1
Khusia	*Hedichium sp.*	29.0	2.3	25.3	39.5	-	-	8.9
Preyano	*Ficus religiosa*	13.6	2.6	16.2	61.2	-	-	6.4
Medzei	*Spondias pinnata*	19.4	2.0	17.8	52.3	-	-	8.5

*g/100g fresh matter; DM dry matter; CP crude protein; EE ether extract; NFE nitrogen free extract; CT condensed tannin

states. 2-3 cuttings can be obtained with an average yield of 60-95 kg/tree/cut. This tree provides the green fodder during the lean period (October to December) for feeding the mithun and other livestock. It is most common the farmer's loppe this tree especially during the October to December when other fodder tree remains dry. It is also named as Kartoos as per the nepali workers.

Conclusion

Lots of information has been generated in the National Research Centre on Mithun, Nagaland and the institute has been trying to popularize the tree leaves and shrubs generally consumed by mithun, their chemical composition and nutritive value. In the future if any tree leaves/shrubs are found to be good for mithun will be popularized among the farmers. The tree leaves/shrubs must be fed as mixture or cocktail either in stall fed condition or in grazing condition for better performance in animals.

Chapter 4

Scientific Feeding Practices for Optimum Swine Production in Rural India

S.K. MONDAL[1] AND S.K. SAHA[2]
[1]Senior Scientist and [2]Senior Scientist, Division of Animal Nutrition
Indian Veterinary Research Institute, Izatnagar, Bareilly - 243 122

Introduction

One of the best meat producing animals in the world is the pig that has high prolificacy with short generation interval, efficient mothering ability, rapid growth, most economic feed conversion efficiency and high dressing percentage. An integrated approach for livestock farming is the key to address the challenges faced by our country in securing the food as well as nutritional security to the fast growing human population. Among the various livestock species, pig is the most potential source of meat production and more efficient feed converters after the broiler. Apart from providing meat, it is also a source of bristles and manure. Pig farming provides quick returns since the marketable weight of fatteners can be achieved within a period of 6-8 months. There is good demand from domestic as well as export market for pig products such as pork, bacon, ham, sausages and lard etc. Pig farming is capable of providing employment opportunities to seasonally employed rural farmers and supplementary income to improve their living standards. Very recently, a dramatic shift towards small to medium-sized commercial pig farming with growing interest in self-employing educated rural Indian youth is being evident.

The pig farming encompasses many farm operations/activities to be put together and feeding is most important among them. Feeding accounts over 75% of the total cost of raising pigs in India. The pigs produce more live weight gain from a given weight of feed than any other class of meat producing animals, but at the same time, they also consume more feed per unit body weight. The pigs can utilize wide variety of feed stuffs viz. grains, forages, damaged feeds and garbage and convert them into valuable nutritious meat. The locally available cheaper feedstuffs can conveniently be blended into pig ration. However, the pigs can be fed with a limited quantity of roughages and feeding of damaged grains, garbage and other unbalanced rations may result in lower feed efficiency.

Characteristic features of Swine

While planning for feeds and feeding of pigs, it is very important to consider the salient features of swine digestive system as well as the metabolic processes involving their better growth and feed conversion efficiency. Some such points are outlined below:

i) Pigs are omnivorous mono-gastric animal with well developed ceacum and colon, so they can consume a wide variety of feeds including kitchen wastes etc. but with a limited quantity of roughage.

ii) Ration must have more concentrates with adequate content of quality protein (amino acids content) and vitamins including B-Complex.

iii) Type of feed and the methods of feeding greatly influence feed efficiency, growth rate, breeding efficiency, carcass quality and the health in general.

iv) Pigs can convert inedible feeds to edible meat, but may sometimes directly compete with human beings for cereals.

v) Pigs are prone to suffer from nutritional deficiencies.

vi) Small pasture with green forages is good for raising pigs.

vii) Three types of rations are fed to pigs before they reach maturity; i.e., creep, grower and finisher.

Problems in supplying feed nutrients to pigs

i) Pigs must be provided with balanced diets with sufficient protein, minerals, vitamins, fats and carbohydrates in their daily ration.

ii) Nutritional deficiencies need proper correction to avoid piglet losses.

iii) Good palatable ration (preferably made of non-conventional feed ingredients) with all essential nutrients must be provided as per age and physiological conditions.

iv) Recommended level of nutrients for swine varies with the age, weight and physiological condition as well as their estimation procedures.

v) Feeding trials on pigs are a must for estimating availability of nutrients in feeds.

vi) The forms of feed stuff also influence the availability of feed nutrients.

vii) Some other factors like stress, nutrient interrelationship, feed additives and subclinical disease level also influence the variation in the requirements and availability of feed nutrients to pigs.

Feeding management

Feed is the most important component that influences the profit from a swine enterprise.

Successful swine production requires a carefully planned and efficient feeding programme. The feed should be selected based on the tendency of pig farming for being more specialized and intensified even in rural areas. Through proper breeding and selection, rapid growing strains of swine have been developed. Owners of the farms now plan to market their hogs a 5 months of age instead of 7-8 months that was a practice a few years ago. Apart from this, planning for large litters (piglets at a time) and for breeding to farrow twice a year forces the swine producers to adopt refined methods of scientific feeding programmes. Some important points to remember while feeding the swine are as following:

a) Feed the animals with best feeds to meet up their nutrient requirements.

b) Give adequate concentrates with quality protein in their daily ration.

c) Provide adequate vitamins and minerals with special emphasis on B-vitamins.

d) Provide adequate clean portable drinking water during all the seasons.

e) Give adequate exercise to the animals, either through paddock or small good quality green pastures.

f) Feeding of colostrum within a short period from birth is a must for the newborn piglets.

g) The feeding of the piglets is more critical and high quality and more fortified diets are needed for feeding them.

h) Before weaning at 6 weeks of age, it is better to provide adequate creep mixture of good quality for increased growth rate.

i) Sufficient quantity of swine grower ration must be provided.

j) Proper feeding of the sows as per their nutritional requirement during pregnancy is utmost important for increased litter size as well as decreased chances of piglet anaemia.

k) The feed requirements of lactating sow vary with the size of the litter, weight, size and age of sow.

l) Conventional feed ingredients like maize, ground nut cake, wheat bran, deoiled soyabean cake can well be used for pig feeding alongwith proper fish meal, mineral and vitamin supplementation.

m) Commercial pig farming should aim at the exploitation of non-conventional feed resources, preferably locally available, viz., waste from kitchen/ hotel/ cold storage/warehouses, in suitably replacing the balanced rations to minimize the cost of production.

n) The feeding regime adopted should take care of all the nutrient requirements of various categories of pigs. The nutrient requirements of growing pigs and breeding stock are given in Tables 1 and 2.

Table 1 : Nutrient requirements of growing pigs

Type	Weaning	Growing	Finishing
Live weight (kg)	5-12	12-50	50-100
Daily gain (kg)	0.3	0.5	0.6
Energy and protein			
DE (Mcal/kg)	3.5	3.5	3.3
ME (Mcal/kg)	3.36	3.36	3.17
Crude Protein (%)	22	18	14
Inorganic nutrients (%)			
Calcium	0.8	0.65	0.5
Phosphorus	0.6	0.5	0.4
Sodium	—	0.1	—
Chlorine	—	0.13	—

Table 2 : Nutrient requirements of breeding stock

Type	Breed Gilts	Lactating gilts and sows	Young boars & adult boars
Live weight (kg.)	110-250	140-250	110-250
Energy and protein			
DE (Mcal/kg)	3.3	3.3	3.3
ME (Mcal/kg)	3.17	3.17	3.17
Crude Protein (%)	14	15	14
Inorganic nutrients (%)			
Calcium	0.75	0.75	0.75
Phosphorus	0.5	0.5	0.5
Salt	0.5	0.5	0.5

Conclusions

Scientific feeding of pigs in rural areas needs a careful insight of the nutrient requirement of the pigs at their different age and physiological condition. The nutritional peculiarities of swine should be considered in positive sense while planning for feeding them with most economic unconventional feed stuff. The deficiencies in relation to nutrition and health problems should be corrected with a promptness to make the swine production enterprise successful. Most economic feed ingredients (locally available non-conventional) and efficient feeding programme are key to success in pig farming business. The problems of feeding pigs should be looked into in totality alongwith other farm planning components like breeding, management and health coverage as they all are interrelated for achieving success in swine production enterprise.

Chapter 5

Emergence of Highly Virulent Avian Influenza in India

S. NANDI
Indian Veterinary Research Institute, Izatnagar, Bareilly - 243122 (U.P.)

Introduction

Avian influenza (AI) earlier known as fowl plaque or fowl pest, a highly contagious and infectious disease of birds, is now popularly known as avian flu or bird flu. All the birds are thought to be vulnerable to avian influenza but poultry chicken, turkeys, quails, guinea fowls etc are more prone to AI virus infection which may reach rapidly to epidemic proportion. Influenza A virus infections in poultry can be divided into two distinct groups on the basis of their ability to cause disease (1) highly pathogenic avian influenza (HPAI) and (2) low pathogenicity avian influenza (LPAI). Influenza viruses have been shown to affect all types of domestic and captive birds in all the areas of the world. But the frequency of primary infections in any type of birds depends on the degree of contact with the feral birds. In 2006, in

Maharashtra, M.P. and Gujarat, in 2007 in Manipur and in 2008 in 13 districts (Birbhum, Murshidabad, South Dinajpur, Burdwan, Nadia, Bankura, Malda, South 24 Paragans, Hooghly, West Midnapur, Howrah, Darjeeling and Coochbehar) of West Bengal were affected with outbreaks of the disease in poultry farms leading to the culling of huge number of birds thus causing enormous economic losses in the pilot industry. Among these 3 consecutive outbreaks in 3 years the outbreaks in W.B. is the most severe and worst one according to WHO affecting 13 out of 19 districts.

Poultry industry in India at a glance : Poultry farming has become a profitable industry in India and has the potential to improve the national economy. India ranks fourth in egg production and fifth in broiler production in the world. The layer industry is growing at the rate of 5-7% against the broiler industry at 10-12% per annum. However, the per capita availability of eggs and broiler meat is far below the ICMR recommended level of 180 eggs and 11 Kg meat per annum. With the present growth rate, by 2010 AD there will be 245 million layers and 2500 million broilers. With a turn over of more than 300 billion rupees, the Indian Poultry Industry (IPI) provides direct and indirect employment to over 5 million people in the country and has great potential to create gainful employment with every increase in egg/meat consumption. It accounts about 1% of the India's gross domestic product (GDP) and 10% of the total GDP attributed to livestock products. If the gap between the availability and requirement is fulfilled, it is likely to create over 10 million jobs.

Considering the world's total production, India's contribution is about 2% chicken and 4% eggs only. In overall market of poultry, India has been positioned 17th in the world poultry production. The value of India's poultry and poultry products production annually stands at Rs 30,000 crore of which the export market is worth just Rs 300 crore. The value of India 's poultry exports between 2005-2006 was at Rs 167.58 crore and Rs 302.02 crore in 2006-07.

Etiology : Influenza viruses belong to the *Orthomyxoviridae* family and either *Influenzavirus A* or *Influenza virus B* or *Influenzavirus C* genus. These viruses are identified by antigenic differences in their nucleoprotein and matrix protein. Influenza A viruses infect mammals and birds whereas influenza B and C viruses infect only humans. These viruses have segmented negative sense single stranded RNA genome enclosed by lipid envelope from which haemagglutinin (H) and neuraminidase (N) polypeptides are projected. Eight pieces of negative sense single stranded RNA are present in influenza A virus and these code for at least ten viral polypeptides which are either incorporated into progeny virus (structural proteins) or are produced in infected cells but not found in virus particles (non-structural proteins). The type A influenza virus is most likely to cause epidemics and pandemics as it can undergo antigenic shift and present a new immune target to susceptible people. Populations tend to have more resistance to influenza B and C because they only undergo antigenic drift and have more similarity with the previous strains. Antigenic shift is the process by which two different strains of influenza virus combine to form a new subtype by exchanging the RNA segments which is characterized by a mixture of the surface antigen of the two original strains whereas antigenic drift refers to point mutations in the influenza virus over time.

Recent outbreaks of avian influenza : Besides the four pandemics of influenza reported in last centuries in 1918 (H1N1), 1957 (H2N2), 1968 (H3N2) and 1977 (H1N1), an unprecendented epizootic of avian influenza A (H5N1) that is highly pathogenic has crossed the species barrier to cause many human fatalities. Person to person transmission of H5N1 was not recognized. A precursor to the 1997 H5N1 strain was identified in Guangdong, China in 1996 when it caused death in geese. H5N1 strains circulate among birds worldwide and are responsible for the current panzootic among domestic poultry and other birds in Asia, Europe and Africa. Since January 2002, the predominant genotype of H5N1 in Southern China has been genotype Z. This genotype then spread into Southeast Asia in 2003, causing severe outbreaks in poultry in Thailand, Cambodia and Vietnam. Since 2005, a sublineage of Z genotype (termed Fujian like or FJ like) has emerged as the predominant variant in Southern China. Recent genetic characterization of H5N1 viruses has demonstrated two distinct phylogenetic clades. Clade 1 viruses have circulated primarily in Cambodia, Thailand and Vietnam and Clade 2 viruses have circulated primarily in China and Indonesia and have spread westward to the Middle East, Europe and Africa. Six different subclades of clade 2 have been recognized. A recent study involving genetic characterization of two H5N1 appears to be expanding its host range, has caused a number of human deaths and the possibility that H5N1 could mutate into a human pandemic strain is causing woıldwide concern.

Characteristics of current avian influenza strain : Studies comparing virus samples over time indicate that the virus is now able to progressively more pathogenic for poultry. The current strain of the virus is now able to survive several days longer in the environment compared to strain emerged initially. The virus appears to be expanding its mammalian host range. The virus has been found increasingly in dead migratory birds which are unusually not clinically affected by HPAI viruses indicates the growing virulence of the current virus. Recent nucleotide sequencing performed on viral isolates from turkey demonstrates that the strains contain two mutations which may make the virus better adapted to humans. These mutations could potentially enhance transmission from birds to humans and between humans. Influenza experts are concerned that if the H5N1 virus reassorts with human influenza viruses a new influenza virus with pandemic potential could emerge. Another possibility is for an avian strain to gradually adapt to the human populations and develop into a pandemic strain without genetic reassortment. For a pandemic to occur the new virus would need to be highly pathogenic for humans and easily transmitted from person to person.

All 84 characterised viruses from Indonesia were belonged to H5N1 clade 2.1 with three virus sublineages being identified: clade 2.1.1 (1), clade 2.1.3 (80), and IDN/6/05-like viruses (3) that did not belong to any of the present clades. All three clades were found in ducks, while only clade 2.1.3 was isolated from chickens. There were no significant amino acid mutations of the haemagglutinin (HA) and neuraminidase (NA) sites of the viruses, including the receptor binding, glycosylation, antigenic and catalytic sites and NA inhibitor targets. All the viruses had polybasic amino acids at the HA cleavage site. No evidence of major antigenic variants was detected. Based on the HA gene, identical virus variants could be found on different farms across the study sites and multiple genetic variants could be isolated from HPAI outbreaks simultaneously or at different time points from single farms. HPAI virus was isolated from both ducks and chickens; however, the proportion of surviving duck cases was considerably higher than in chickens. The 2.1.3 clade was the most common lineage found. All the viruses had sequence characteristic of HPAI but negligible variations in other recognised amino acids at the HA and NA proteins which determine virus phenotypes. Multiple genetic variants appeared to be circulating simultaneously within poultry communities. It was noted that the high proportion of live duck cases compared to chickens over the study period suggests that ducks are more likely to survive infection and they may better suit the role of long-term maintenance host for H5N1. As some viruses were isolated from dead birds, there was no clear correlation between genetic variations and pathogenicity of these viruses.

CDC has been watching the evolution of all H5N1 viruses closely. Changes in viruses that WHO and CDC look for specifically are those that could increase the threat to human health. There is nothing to indicate that clade 2.3.2.1 viruses pose any greater threat to human health than any of the other H5N1 viruses. The clade 2.3.2.1 viruses are very active viruses and are spreading more widely in poultry and wild birds. While this increases the possibility of human exposures to infected birds or poultry, it does not increase their ability to infect and transmit between people. However, as part of the U.S. government's pandemic preparedness activities, a 2.3.2.1 vaccine virus candidate to protect humans against this virus already has been created so that vaccine production could begin rapidly if this virus were to change to infect humans and spread easily from person to person. The vaccine virus candidate is an exact match to currently circulating 2.3.2.1 viruses.

Recent mortality in crows due to birdflu in India : The Indian Government has sent an alert to the Jharkhand government to remain cautious about a possible poultry infection, after a mysterious bird flu-like virus is believed to have killed between 500 and 1,000 crows in Jamshedpur, Ranchi, Bokaro, Khuti, Sahebganj, parts of Hazaribagh and other districts of the state. A study on the crow deaths conducted at the High security Animal Disease Laboratory in Bhopal found a virus resembling that of bird flu and the virus was detected only in the brain of the dead crows. The strain is different from the one that had infected poultry in Maharashtra some years ago. It is for the first time that it has been found in the country. The strain has been compared with the strains isolated in Vietnam, Indonesia and other places in Asia and found similarities with the Vietnam strain. The virus was not found in the fecal matter or esophageal swabs of the dead crows. This means it cannot spread from one crow to another or any other bird unless the flesh of an infected crow is consumed by another scavenger. A team of scientists from the Indian Veterinary Research Institute had visited Jamshedpur to collect samples of crow carcasses and made prima facie observations. The symptoms shown by the infected crows include quivering, high body temperatures and convulsions.

Bird flu was detected in crow too in Orissa at Keranga in Khurda district and Angul after test at High Security Animal Disease Laboratory (HSADL) in Bhopal. Meanwhile culling of fowls got underway in tribal dominated Mayurbhanj, the second district in the state hit by avian influenza. Death of a large number of crows and other birds in different areas of the state including Jagatsinghpur, Paradip, Mayurbhanj, Dhenkanal and Sundargarh had also been reported. The animal husbandry department had culled 8,500 fowls in over 20 villages in Bahanada area. Twenty rapid response teams were engaged in culling.

Virus and the disease : Influenza A viruses infecting poultry birds can be divided into two distinct groups on the basis of their ability to cause disease in chickens. The very virulent viruses called highly pathogenic avian influenza (HPAI) or bird flu in which mortality may be as high as 100%. These viruses have been restricted to subtypes H5 and H7, although most of the viruses of these subtypes cause only low pathogenicity avian influenza (LPAI) and only a few percentages of all H5 and H7 subtypes of AI viruses cause HPAI. All the other subtypes of AI viruses have been reported in the majority of possible combinations from the birds and cause only LPAI. It is to be noted that the two H10 subtype (H10N4 and H10N5) of influenza A viruses have also been reported to be fulfilling the criteria given by OIE and EU of becoming the HPAI.

The HPAI can cause serious infections in some species of birds on a farm while leaving others unaffected. The clinical signs are variable. The typical symptoms are sinusitis, lacrymation, oedema of head, cyanosis of the head, comb and wattle and green to white diarrhea. Haemorrhagic lesions are observed on the comb and wattle of turkeys. Anorexia, coughing, sneezing, blood tinged oral and nasal discharge, ecchymoses on the shanks of feet, neurological symptoms and reduced egg production, loss of egg pigmentation and deformed or shell less eggs are also commonly observed signs. Sudden death may occur with other symptoms. Most of the flock usually dies. In ducks, the most common symptoms are sinusitis, diarrhea and increased mortality.

The low pathogenic avian influenza (LPAI) viruses usually cause subclinical or mild illness. The symptoms may include decreased egg production, mild to moderate respiratory disease and low mortality rate (5%). More severe disease mimicking highly pathogenic avian influenza with high mortality (up to 50%) may also be seen in birds infected with LPAI when the condition is aggravated due to presence of secondary bacterial infection or other intercurrent viral diseases.

Most of the AI infections do not produce any recognizable disease in free living or wild birds. All these birds are the asymptomatic reservoirs of the AI viruses. Wild waterfowl and other aquatic birds (ducks, geese, shorebirds, gulls, swans, terns) are the reservoir of all AI viruses. Natural infections of wild birds with HPAI are rare. Viruses of H5 or H7 subtypes isolated from the free living birds are almost invariably of low pathogenicity for poultry. Seasonal coming of migratory waterfowls may allow the regular addition of new viruses to the diverse domestic poultry virus pool in the backyard poultry system.

Lesions : HPAI in poultry birds may cause oedematous, haemorrhagic and necrotic lesions in skin and visceral organs namely lungs, spleen, heart, liver, kidney, pancreas etc. Petechial haemorrhages of whole viscera and peritoneum with generalized congestion are observed. Histologically, multiorgan necrosis and/or inflammation occurs. Brain, heart, lung and pancreas along with primary and secondary lymphoid organs are most severely affected. There is perivascular cuffing of lymphocytes in brain, heart, spleen and pancreas, coagulative necrosis in kidney, lungs and spleen, haemorrhagic streaks in heart muscles with focal degeneration to necrosis, urate casts in kidney tubules, lymphocytic meningoencephalitis with focal gliosis and neuronal necrosis. Necrosis, apoptosis and depletion of lymphocytes are common in the bursa, thymus and spleen.

LPAI in poultry birds may produce lesions in respiratory tract especially the sinusitis and tracheitis with thickened mucous and catarrhal, fibrinous and mucopurulent inflammation. The tracheal mucosa can be oedematous with congestion and haemorrhages. Microscopically there is diffused pneumonia, heterophilic to lymphocytic tracheitis and bronchitis, nephrosis and nephritis, pancreatitis, lymphocyte depletion and apoptosis of lymphocytes in the bursa, thymus and spleen.

References

Capua, I. and Alexander, D.J. (2002). Avian influenza and human health. Acta Trop. 83 (11) :1-6.

Fleming, D. (2005). Influenza pandemics and avian flu. British Med. J. 331 :1066-1069.

Horimoto, T. and Kawaoka, Y. (2005). Influenza : lesions from past pandemics, warning from current incidents. Nat. Rev. Microbiol. 3(8) : 591-600.

Hulse, D. J. et al. (2005). Role of domestic ducks in the propagation and biological evolution of highly pathogenic H5N1 influenza viruses in Asia. Proc. Natl. Acad. Sci. USA. 102 (30) : 10682-10687.

Katx, J.M. (2003). The impact of avian influenza on public health. Avian Disease. 47 : 914-920.

Nandi, D., Hajra, S. and Nandi, S. 2006. Bird flu – a scourge to poultry industry. Poultryline, 6:4: 15-18.

Nandi, S. 2004. Avian influenza – a threat to poultry industry. Indian Farming, 54: 4 : 30-32.

Padhi, S., Panigrathi, P.K., Mahapatra, A. and Mahapatra, S. (2004). Avian influenza A (H5N1) : a preliminary review. Indian J. Medical Microbiol. 22:3:143-146.

Perdue, M.L. and Swayne, D.E. (2005). Public health risk from avian influenza viruses. Avian Disease. 49 (3) : 317-327.

Perdue, M.L., Suarez, D. L. and Swayne, D.E. (1999). Avian influenza in the 1990s. Poultry and Avian Biology Reviews. 11 : 1-20.

Reid A.H., Tau ben berger, J. K. and Fanning, T.G.(2001). The 1918 Spanish influenza : integrating history and biology. 3: 81-87.

Shortridge, K. F. (1992). Pandemic influenza : a zoonosis. Semin Respir. Infect. 7:11-25.

Shortridge, K.F. (1999). Poultry and the influenza H5N1 outbreak in Hong Kong, 1997 : abridged chronology and virus isolation. Vaccine. 17 : 526-529.

Suarez, D.L. et al., (1998). Comparison of highly virulent H5N1 influenza A viruses isolated from humans and chickens in Hong Kong. J. Virol. 72 : 6678-6688.

Webby, R.J., and Webster, R.G. (2003). Are we ready for pandemic influenza. Science. 203 :1519-1521.

Yuen, K. Y. et al., (1998). Clinical features and rapid viral diagnosis of human disease associated with avian influenza A H5N1 virus. Lancet. 351 : 467-471.

Yuen, K. Y. et al., (1998). Clinical features and rapid viral diagnosis of human disease associated with avian influenza A H5N1 virus. Lancet. 351 : 467-471.

□□□

Chapter 6

Designing Poultry Meat and Eggs through Dietary Approaches

A.B. MANDAL AND PRAVIN K. TYAGI
Central Avian Research Institute, Izatnagar, Bareilly - 243 122 (U.P.)

The poultry industry in India has emerged as dynamic and fast growing segment in animal husbandry sector with an annual growth rate of 6 to 19% in broiler chickens and 5-7% in egg production during 1980 - 2010. The productivity and feed utilization efficiency of meat-type chickens and eggs have also improved dramatically due to the concomitant progress in improvement of genetic make-up, rearing methods, nutrition and feeding management, disease prevention, medication and bio-security. Poultry industry, being most organized one has the potential to solve the malnutrition and unemployment problems and augment rural economy in a state where in agricultural production has reached nearly to a plateau. The present society is very much concerned on clean and safe environment besides animal welfare and production of safe products akin to customers demand. The poultry products like meat and eggs by default have already gained a healthy image. Moreover, efforts are also being made to design these produce to perform a particular function or set of functions effectively and reliably, to suit the purposes and the attitudes of the consumers. With the self-sufficiency and adequate levels of quantitative food production, increasing capacity of purchasing power of consumers with more earnings, change in life style, and public demand for food of specific quality and purpose, the quality and designing aspects have got emphasis in many developed and underdeveloped countries. In the integrated production system, designer products may play an important role in providing additional profit to the producers, if quality commands premium price in a given market. Though, India is still deficient in quantitative supply to meet the demand of the poultry products, but designing aspects can also be exploited for improving long-term market prospects. Moreover, in the competitive market, who respond successfully remains always gainer. Again such designing provides scope for enjoying delicacy and taste to the consumers especially afraid of taking conventional eggs and meat for different health reason.

Improving consumers' health and nutritional status by designing nutritional profile of poultry meat and eggs through dietary approaches is relatively simple concept.

Nutrition of birds influences meat qualities in terms of nutritive value, acceptability, human health and processing. Similarly, eggs can be designed through dietary approaches either through feed intrinsic factors, supplementation of specific nutrients or certain herbs or specific drugs. Designing eggs is important as the per capita egg consumption in world is decreasing due to presence of high cholesterol and problems associated with Salmonella in eggs. Moreover, eggs can be enriched with certain specific nutrients or agents that have functional and therapeutic properties.

Dietary approaches for designer meat

The major changes in meat that can be brought through nutritional manipulation are increase in protein with concomitant decrease in fat and cholesterol, enrichment of meat with specific fatty acids, fat-soluble vitamins and probably certain minerals. The chemical composition of white and red meat is different. The white meat contains 74.41% moisture, 23.40% protein, 0.80% fat, 1.14% ash, 0.005% calcium and 0.273% phosphorus, while red meat contains 75.26% moisture, 19.11% protein, 4.12% fat, 1.04% ash, 0.005% calcium and 0.186% phosphorus. Breast meat was 21.94% of live body weight and breast meat gain to mass of cut carcass is about 29.7%, while leg and thigh meat to live weight was lower at

15.57%, while the leg and thigh meat to cut carcass weight is 21%. Manipulating energy to protein ratio and amino acid concentration in diets can increase the breast yield, and relative concentration of protein and moisture in breast and thigh muscles.

There are growing public concern over consumption of poultry meat having more cholesterol and saturated fatty acids. Coronary heart disease and arterioscelorosis are strongly related to the dietary intake of cholesterol and saturated fatty acids. Chicken meat is relatively low in fat and cholesterol, and thus considered healthier than other animal protein sources. Numerous including dietary factors have been demonstrated to alter fat deposition and cholesterol contents in meat. Dietary supplementation of methionine; lysine, glycine, tryptophan, amino acid mixtures and chromium can reduce body fat deposition. Dietary fiber also reduces fat concentration and facilitates lean meat production. Dehydrated alfalfa is a good source of hypocholesterolaemic compounds such as saponins. Dietary supplementation of garlic, copper and omega-3 fatty acids has been used successfully to reduce cholesterol content in poultry meat. Supplementation of Cu (35 to 126 mg/kg feed) increases oleic acid content and reduces meat cholesterol. Different probiotics in diet have been reported to improved moisture, protein, ash, and decrease fat and cholesterol content in leg and breast meat of chickens.

The omega-3 group of polyunsaturated fatty acids (PUFA) has received attention from health professionals and nutritionists in recent past due to their beneficial effect on human health. Higher intake of PUFA decreases the risk of heart diseases and strokes, and also exerts immunological and neurological effects and has positive effects in the prevention of heart beat irregularities, cancers, aging and even depression, and improving blood lipid profile and blood coagulation. The (decosahexaenoic acid) DHA is a major component of brain tissues and retina. Its intake is positively correlated in learning process and deficiency is related to impaired retinal function. Broiler chicken is an excellent alternative source of PUFA. Many studies are also being directed towards the manipulation of the fatty acid composition of broiler chicks further to augment human health. The main sources of PUFA are fish oil, linseed, millets and sea algae. The sea algae are the best sources to enrich meat with omega-3 fatty acid. Moreover, the PUFA of algae origin are more stable and in more active form than that in plant oils. Certain cereals like corn, barley and oats are also rich in linolenic acid. The combination of animal (fish) and vegetable (rapeseed, linseed) oils are also effective. Enrichment in n-3 fatty acids results in higher rate of oxidation that could be controlled by the antioxidants such as alpha-tocopherol or vitamin E.

Conjugated linoleic acids (CLA) are the natural components of animal foods derived from linoleic acid, also have been proved as beneficial. Numerous health beneficial effects have been attributed to CLA in experimental animal models over the past two decades that include ameliorating carcinogenesis, atheroscelerosis, onset of diabetes and body fat mass or obesity. CLA is also a potent regulator of body fat accumulation and retention.

Intestinal colonization of Salmonella, Campylobacter and Coliforms in the chickens is the source of contamination in carcass during slaughter. Salmonella and Campylobacter cause gastro-enteritis in human beings. Nutritional manipulation that affects colonization of these bacteria may reduce their contamination in carcass. Feeding of different probiotics and prebiotics, and pre-slaughter fasting hour also influences microbiological meat quality.

Poultry meat is highly susceptible to oxidative rancidity or lipid oxidation during frozen storage. Lipid oxidation is a complex process that accounts for the appearance of rancidity during fresh meat storage and causes the development of warmed-over flavours when cooked meat is stored or reheated. Moreover, the oxidative stability of cholesterol is also less. It is easily converted to oxidative products in presence of light and molecular oxygen, which are potent carcinogen and atherogen. Similarly the unsaturated fatty acids are also susceptible to oxidative rancidity. The process is believed to begin at the cellular membrane level and particularly affects the polyunsaturated fatty acids and cholesterol resulting in loss of membrane integrity and generation of compounds affecting the flavour, colour, and texture of the meat, nutritive value of meat and the acceptability of the product by the consumer. The oxidation of unsaturated lipids leads to formation of hydroperoxides as the primary products which are then broken down to produce volatile and nonvolatile compounds. Volatile compounds are related to acceptability or rejection of food products, while the nonvolatile compounds mainly affect the safety of the consumers as oxidative stress is involved in the pathology of cancer, arteriosclerosis, malaria, and rheumatoid arthritis and plays a role in neurodegenerative diseases and aging process. The cells have protective agents that guard against damage induced by oxygen reactive species. The enzymes glutathione peroxidase, catalase, superoxide dismutase constitute an antioxidant cellular enzyme system.

Naturally occurring antioxidant - vitamin E or alfa-tocopherol had been reported to be effective in improving self-life of poultry meat and meat products through delaying lipid oxidation. Thigh meat is more susceptible to lipid oxidation than breast meat (about 22% of live body weight or 30% of carcass mass). The oxidative stability of poultry meat is related to tissue concentration of tocopherol. As the level of vitamin E in diet increases there is concomitant increase in its concentration in tissues and having following order of deposition in descending order: egg yolk, liver, adipose tissue and muscle. Higher levels of vitamin E in poultry not only improve the oxidative stability but also prevent excessive drip loss. The sensory quality of meat assessed from scoring of aroma, flavour, taste, etc. is reported to be improved by adding vitamin E in diets of broilers. Even vitamin E decreases the production of fishy flavour because of fishmeal oil supplementation in diet and warmed over flavour in refrigerated cooked meat and raw frozen meat. For poultry, levels of 7mg/kg α-tocopherol in muscle are recommended to prolong the keeping quality of meat.

The role of dietary selenium (Se) in influencing the quality of poultry meat and meat products appears to have not been studied to a great extent so far. Nevertheless, based on the knowledge of Se deficiency conditions in poultry, which causes exudative diathesis and muscular dystrophy, it is possible to assume that Se (glutathione peroxidase) may have a significant role on the quality of poultry meat and meat products. Supplementation of vitamin A, methionine, oregano, rosemary essential oils, astaxanthin and lasalacid sodium salt may also be beneficial for improving oxidative stability of meat under cold chain.

Dietary approaches for designer eggs

The eggs have been described as "Nature's original functional food" (packed with all the important vitamins and minerals, except vitamin C. The quality of egg protein is also considered better than many animal protein sources. Eggs are also the cheapest sources of quality nutritional package. One large egg contributes about 70-80 kcal of energy, 7 g of protein, total fat 4.5 g, saturated fat 1.5 g, polyunsaturated fat 0.5g, monounsaturated fat 2.0 g, cholesterol 200-250 mg, sodium 65 mg, potassium 60 mg, total carbohydrate 1 g, choline (300 mg) and significant quantity of vitamin B12, folate, selenium, riboflavin, vitamin D, phosphorus, vitamin E and vitamin A. The nutritive composition can be altered through dietary approaches. Consumers can now find eggs with less cholesterol and saturated fat than conventional one with additional vitamin E and omega-3 fatty acids as bonus.

Egg yolk is the excellent, highly bio-available source of the carotenoids, lutein and zeaxanthin. Recent research demonstrated the link between these dietary compounds and the macular pigment of the retina of the eye. Lutein and zeaxanthin are the primary carotenoids found in the mascular region. Sufficient quantities of these nutrients in the diet are thought to reduce the risk of age-related mascular degeneration, a leading cause of old-age blindness. Besides reducing the risk of mascular degeneration, lutein has a protective effect for early atherosclerosis. Increased amounts of dietary lutein from green leafy vegetables and egg yolks could help in protecting against atherosclerosis by slowing the progression of atherosclerotic lesions in humans and animals. Early atherosclerosis was inversely related to levels of plasma lutein which were affected by dietary intake indicating an inverse relationship between dietary lutein and atherosclerosis development.

To cater the growing demands of health conscious consumers, the eggs are being designed but yet a small percentage of eggs are sold as designer eggs. The possibilities for designing eggs are limitless. The eggs may be designed for enhanced nutritionally, value addition and added processing. Free range eggs are produced by hens that are not kept in cages. Hens have daily access to outdoors, depending on the climate. The nutrient content of free-range eggs is identical to conventional eggs provided not kept in different feeding regimen. Organic eggs are produced by hens kept under the norms of organic farming. The eggs produced from hen fed completely vegetarian diet are generally termed as vegetarian eggs suitable for lacto-ovo-vegetarians. Eggs marketed with low cholesterol or modified fat, contains less cholesterol, less saturated fat, more omega-

3 fatty acids and vitamin E in comparison to conventional generic shell eggs. The cholesterol and saturated fat contents can be reduced to an extent of about 30% through dietary manipulations. Linolenic acid is the major acid in egg yolk. The egg yolk is a good vehicle for DHA, arachidonic acid and EPA. The hens fed diets or feedstuffs (linseed oil, fish oil, etc.) containing high in omega-3 fatty acids produce eggs with high omega-3 fatty acid content in the yolks. Similarly, enrichment of diet of with iodine or vitamin E increases their concentration in eggs. The hens fed herbs, garlic or higher copper in diet had eggs with low cholesterol. About 35% reduction in cholesterol contents of eggs has been possible.

Lutein is a xanthophyll carotenoid present in dark green leaves, leaf meal, leafy vegetables, corn gluten meal and egg yolk. These are widely distributed in tissues and are the principal carotenoids in the eye lens and mascular region of the retina. It has potential for the prevention of numerous diseases in human. An inverse relationship was reported based on epidemiological studies between xanthophyll intake or its status in the body and cataract as well as age-related mascular degeneration. Moreover, these xanthophylls may help in reducing the risk of certain types of cancer (particularly those of the breast and lung) and prevention of heart disease and stroke. There is also role of lutein and zeaxanthin in disease prevention. The lutein content in eggs is directly correlated with the lutein concentration in hens diet.

Designer meat and eggs provide options for consumers who want those products with different nutritional benefits than generic eggs. With the advent of more knowledge on interaction of different dietary intrinsic (nutrients) and extrinsic factors (herbs/drugs) on the quality of eggs and meat in terms of nutritive value, acceptability, human health aspects, processing, etc. it seems that the dietary approaches will be a safe and user-friendly tool for designing eggs and meat. The major changes that can be brought in meat and egg through nutritional manipulation are increase of protein with concomitant decrease in fat, enrichment of meat with fatty acids, fat-soluble vitamins and probably certain minerals. Numerous nutritional and non-nutritional factors have been demonstrated to alter fat deposition and cholesterol contents in meat and egg. Such designing will help to remove phobia for high cholesterol and fat and thus will certainly help in increasing consumption of poultry products. Moreover, the heart patients will have scope for enjoying delicious poultry meat and eggs. However, designer poultry products should be produced economically, salable profitably, and safe for human consumption. Designing must take into consideration the particular production facilities, available materials, know-how, and economic resources of the producers. Moreover, the welfare aspects and production potentiality of birds and environmental issues must also be taken care of in the process of designer eggs and meat.

Chapter 7

Diagnostic Approach to the Infection of Mammary Glands - An Overview

SHRIKANT KATOLE, RAVINDRA JADHAV, PRARABDH BADGUJAR, K.L.KHURANA AND AJIT KUMAR

Indian Veterinary Research Institute, Izatnagar, Bareilly – 243 122 (U.P.)

Mastitis is the inflammation of the mammary gland in response to bacterial infection (Wu *et. al.*, 2007). Dairy industry is the most affected by infection of mammary gland and is a major global problem in dairy sector. India ranks first in milk production in terms of quantity but the quality of milk remains a concern. Mastitis is most devastating disease of dairy animals and accounts for huge losses to the farmers as well as to the nation in terms of economic return (Varshney and Naresh, 2005; Christy and Thiruna-vukkarasu, 2006). An estimated annual economic loss of Rs. 2646 crores due to mastitis is reported (Dua, 2001). Extensive research has been conducted and being carried out across the globe on prevention, control and treatment of mastitis. But, till date problem is not under control despite of various measures. Further, Locatelli *et al.*

(2010) reported control measures to a control and monitoring of the spreading of resistant bacterial strains and of the genes responsible for mastitis. More than 100 different types of microbes have been found to be causative agents for mastitis in various animals. Bacteria are the major pathogens of mastitis. Main culprits are *Staphylococcus, Streptococcus* and *E. coli*. Early diagnosis of mastitis pays better in the form of quick therapy in initial stages of disease which gives better results than delayed treatment due to late diagnosis of mastitis.

Visible changes in milk are the most important criteria's to detect the disease, like change in color, consistency, yield etc. Milk may be off color, watery, bloody or have the appearance of serum. Abnormal milk may also contain varying amounts of pus and clots, depending upon the type of infection. The degree of swelling, severity of pain and the overall physiological picture of the udder will indicate the severity of infection and serve as a guide for the course of treatment. General gross symptoms seen are swelling and reddening of mammary glands. Of all the efforts, proper diagnosis of mastitis is the most important aspect to prescribe proper medication. Diagnosis of subclinical infection is more problematic since the infected milk appears normal but usually has an elevated somatic cell count, which can be judged by Somatic Cell Count (SCC). In such case, milk culture will indicate the presence of mastitis pathogens but will not provide visible clinical symptoms associated with the clinical case of mastitis. Much of the literature is available illustrating the pathological, medicinal, physiological, nutritional aspect of mastitis. Present article highlights on the diagnostic aspects of few methods for easy and early detection of mastitis.

1. Gross examination of mammary gland

Mammary gland should be examined for any abnormality in structural anatomy. The clinical findings of mastitis include abnormalities of secretion, size, consistency and temperature of the mammary gland (Radostits, 2005). Acute disease is characterised by diffused swelling of the mammary gland accompanied by heat, pain and abnormalities in milk secretion. Gangrene or abscesses may be noted in severe cases of acute mastitis. In severe cases cow resists the touch which signify acute pain.

2. pH

Increase in sodium, potassium, lactose ion causes alkalinity of the mastitic milk which can be judged simply by pH paper strip or pH meter. This test is very simple and easy to perform. Milk from drying off cow is alkaline and will give test positive. Thus, the test has limited use in drying off cow or in late lactation.

3. Methylene blue test

The dye, methylene blue has high redox potential; this ability can be used to find the presence of microorganisms in milk samples. When milk sample is incubated (37ºC), aerobic microorganisms utilize oxygen which results in fading of dye. The time is noted and severity of infection is judged.

In this test, 1 ml of methylene dye is taken in test tube to which 10 ml of milk sample is added, mixed well and incubate at 37ºC, observed for any reduction in color of the dye, which is indicative of the infection.

4. Hotis-Miller test

This test is based on formation of canary yellow colonies of microbes along the sides of test tubes. Chemical used is bromocresol purple. Canary yellow color is indicative of *Streptococcus agalactiae,* whereas, sometimes reddish brown color may develop which suggests *Staphylococcus aureus* infection. This test is named after Hotis and Miller, inventor of this test.

In this test 9.5 ml of milk is taken in test tube and 0.5 ml of bromocresol purple is added, mixed well and incubated for 24 hours at 38ºC and observed for any color formation along the sides of test tube.

5. Strip cup test

Milk from four quarters is taken in a strip cup and observed for gross abnormalities like discoloration, clots, flakes, pus etc. Discoloration in the milk might be seen in the form of blood staining. This procedure gives an early diagnosis of mastitis. Change of normal milk to wateriness is characteristic cases of chronic mastitis. When quarter is lactating, clots and flakes are suggestive of severe degree of inflammation. Flakes at the end of milking imply the presence of tuberculosis (Radostits, 2005).

The normal physiological changes which occur in milk from start of parturition to drying off should be differentiated from pathological changes to minimize suspicion/doubt of the infection.

6. Whiteside test

This is simple and indirect test to detect the mastitic milk. For this test, glass slide with back side painted black should be taken. Place 4-5 drops of milk sample on glass slide and add 2-4 drops of 4% sodium hydroxide (1N NaOH), mixed well or stir rapidly for 30 seconds and spread over the glass slide in a circular fashion. If milk sample along with reagent appears thick and viscid, it indicates acute form of mastitis. In chronic cases, white flakes are found. No such abnormality is found in normal milk.

Intensity of reaction on glass slide is then well correlates with total leukocyte count.

7. California Mastitis Test (CMT)

California mastitis test (CMT) - routinely used for rapid diagnosis of mastitis (Schalm and Noorlander, 1957). The California Mastitis Test is a simple, inexpensive, rapid screening test for mastitis. CMT is most common and popular test for preliminary screening of mastitis in commercial dairy farms. This test is easy to perform and does not require sophisticated instruments to carry out. The test is based upon the amount of cellular nuclear protein present in the milk sample. Mastitic milk shows increased cell number, when CMT reagent reacts with milk, cells gets ruptured and DNA comes out to forms a gel with reagent, which can be detected easily. Since inflammatory cells associated with mastitis are the predominant cell types present in infected milk, the CMT reflects the somatic cell count (SCC) level quite accurately and is a reliable indicator of the severity of infection. This test helps to correlates the CMT score with that of SCC which gives confirmative diagnosis of mastitis (Table 1).

Table 1 : Correlation between CMT score with Somatic Cell Count

CMT Score	Somatic Cell Count Range
Normal (0)	0-200000
Trace infection (1)	200000-400000
Weak infection (2)	400000-12000000
Distinct infection (3)	1200000-5000000
Heavy/strong infection (4 and 5)	Above 5000000

The appropriateness or value of CMT evaluation of bulk milk decreases as herd size increases. The test is appropriate for cow-side evaluation of udder health. By this test farmers could get quick diagnosis and go for treatment without much delay which otherwise results in progression of infection. Collect 3-4 ml of milk from each quarter in CMT paddle after discarding few streams. Add equal volume of CMT reagent and mix immediately with circular motion. The reaction should be graded based on intensity of gel formation and color changes. Grade, description and score for milk sample by CMT is given in table 2.

Table 2 : Grade, description and point score of milk by CMT

Normal	CMT grade	Description
Trace (T)	Slime formation which disappears with paddle movement	1
Weak (+)	Distinct slime, but no gel formation slight purplish color	2
Distinct positive (++)	Viscous with gel formation adherent to the margin of the cup with color changes	3
Strong positive (+++)	The gel form convex projection, the gel does not dislodge after swirling movement of paddle	4 and 5

The CMT has a number of practical uses. In many herds this test is used to screen fresh cows and cows at dry off. This information is useful for selecting cows for further evaluation by milk culture, culling, selective dry cow treatment or extended therapy.

Attention should be given to farmer's complaint that, the certain percentage (10-20%) of cows sampled for bacterial culture based on CMT score will have no bacterial growth. This is due to a number of factors, including short lived infections that have been cleared by the cow or infections that are characterized by intermittent shedding of bacteria e.g. *Streptococcus agalactiae, Staphylococcus aureus* and *Mycoplasma spp.* or mastitis due to physical injury to mammary gland. It is not recommended that CMT results alone be used for immediate treatment unless the specific pathogen is known or is performed in accordance with a treatment protocol recommended by the qualified Veterinarian. Numerous studies have indicated that intensive drug therapy without prior knowledge of any pathogens present in udder is uneconomical and harmful to dairy animals as well as human beings. This is due to the prevalence of resistant infections such as *Staphylococcus aureus, mycoplasma spp., Listeria spp.* and many other environmental infections that respond poorly to treatment during lactation. This may be attributed to extensive use of medicines without prior knowledge of pharmacokinetics and pharmacodynamics of drugs. The CMT can be used to monitor udder health trends over time. Recording individual cow scores on a monthly basis can be a very effective monitoring system that is particularly appropriate for smaller herds. This can be used as a guideline for many other farms.

Cows in first week after calving or in the last stage of lactation may give a strong positive CMT reaction.

8. Anti trypsin level in milk

Milk anti trypsin activity is mainly due to leakage of á-1-protease inhibitor into milk. Concentration of trypsin increases by many folds in milk from infected animal. Limitations to this test are that high levels of anti trypsin are seen in colostrums milk which decreased within few days post calving.

Colorimetric method of determination of anti trypsin activity is also available in which chemical compound (N-benzoylarginine-p-nitroanilide) is used as a substrate. The concentration of trypsin activity measured spectrophotometrically at 405 nm, comparisons and interpolations should be done with standard curves.

9. Electrical Conductivity

Milk electron conductivity is a screening test. Generally, milk from infected animals has a higher electrical conductivity than the normal milk. This is due to tissue damage and the subsequent increase in sodium and chloride ions in milk which results in higher conductivity of electric current. Now-a-days, conductivity sensors are being incorporated in many automated milking systems at well organized farms. The change in electrical conductivity of milk is one of the earliest manifestations associated with new infections making the early detection and recording of suspicious animals. The electrical conductivity of about 5.4 - 5.6 millisiemens/cm (mS/cm) is the reference value for healthy milk samples. More than this value indicates infection of mammary gland.

The greatest trouble associated with this new technology is the sensitivity and specificity of electrical conductivity among herds. Recent advances in this technology in determining herd specific conductivity threshold levels have increased the worth of this screening method in many herds. A positive indication of increased electrical conductivity in a specific animal is an indication for further clinical evaluation of that particular animal for temperature, udder examination, bacterial culture etc. and not generally a signal for immediate treatment. Hand held conductivity meters are now available and may be useful for routine screening animals and inexpensive also.

10. HyMast test

HyMast test is used to differentiate gram negative and gram positive microorganisms. It is a rapid bacteriological test system which has been promoted as a device to assist the Veterinarians to select the appropriate drug therapy for clinical mastitis. The test consists of a plastic vial with a screw-top cap that has a paddle attached. The paddle is embedded with different types of selective growth media on each side. Bacterial growth on one side of the paddle indicates the presence of gram positive i.e. *Staphylococci*, *Streptococci* organisms, whereas growth on the other side indicates the presence of gram negative i.e. *Coliform* organisms.

Milk sample from an aseptically collected quarter or composite is placed in the vial, and the paddle/cap is replaced. The vial is inverted and rotated 2 - 3 times so that the milk completely covers the culture media on both sides of the paddle. The milk is discarded (or saved in a vial for further diagnostic bacteriology, if necessary), and the cap loosely replaced to allow air to enter the vial. The entire test vial is incubated up to 36 hours (38ºC). The operator checks the paddles for bacterial growth at 8 to 12 hour intervals.

The sensitivity and specificity of the test for identifying gram positive organisms is 0.80 and 0.76, respectively. The sensitivity and specificity for identifying gram negative organisms is 0.60 and 0.98, respectively (Leslie et al., 1995).

Uses of the HyMast Milk Bacteriological Test System

- *Clinical mastitis decision making*: The HyMast test can be used in a decision-making protocol to selective target therapy towards gram-positive organisms.

- *Udder health biosecurity*: The HyMast test may be used as a preliminary bacteriological screening test prior to introducing purchased animals into the herd.
- Evaluating the success of dry cow management and therapy programs: In herds with concerns about the rate of new intramammary infections during the dry period, the HyMast test may provide a useful system to evaluate the effectiveness of the dry cow management program. Similarly, concerns about the success of therapy during lactation can be evaluated using the HyMast test to culture samples.

11. NAGase test

N-acetyl-β-D-glucosaminidase (NAGase) is cell associated enzyme and level of this enzyme increases in mastitis due to the influx of leucocytes in mammary gland. Measurement of NAGase enzyme in the milk is reputed to be the best method of detection of mastitis (Radostits, 2005). Substrate used is 4-methylumbelliferyl-N-â-D-glucosaminide, and fluorescent product 4-umbelliferone is then measured at 635 nm. Results are presented in micromoles (mm)/min/ml of milk. NAGase enzyme activity in milk is high at start and end of the lactation.

12. Catalase test

Catalase is present in cells of normal as well as infected milk, but concentration is more in infected milk. Principle of this test is based on release of reactive oxygen species form hydrogen peroxide (H_2O_2) by enzyme catalase. In inflammatory condition activity of catalase enzyme is increased which in indicative of infection of mammary glands indirectly.

13. Bulk milk culture

Bulk tank cultures results are not only reflection of the pathogens present in mastitic herd but also identify those organisms which may contaminate teats of cows, milking environment or milking equipment. For this is a reason it can also be used to evaluate milk quality, milking methods, procedures and overall level of hygiene of milk collection and storage in the farm. Sampling for bulk tank milk is an easy, economical means of determining the presence of mastitic pathogens in a herd.

14. Bacterial isolation

Direct bacterial cultural examination of milk is useful for accurate diagnosis of mastitis and identification of causative organisms which helps in clear understanding of etio-pathogenesis (Dhana and Sethi, 1962). Bacteriological method is gold standard for therapeutic studies (Gentle and Thompson, 1990).

The bacteriological isolation procedures should be carried out under strict sterile environment in laminar flow (Bio-safety cabinet). The identification of causative organism in collected milk samples should be carried out by inoculating 10 μl of milk on 5% bovine blood agar plates with a sterile 'L' shaped loop (Griffin et al., 1977). The causative organisms in the milk samples after incubation at 37ºC for 24 hr should be identified on the basis of colony morphology, hemolytic pattern and smell on 5% blood agar as per norms of International Dairy Federation (1997), gram staining and culture on selective media.

15. Somatic Cell Count Test (SCC)

Somatic cell count (SCC) primarily estimates the polymorphonuclear granulocytes (PMNs), lymphocytes, macrophages and epithelial cells (Lee *et. al.,* 1980). It is an effective tool for diagnosis of mastitis and to assess the severity of damage (Hicks *et al.*, 1994). Somatic cell counts are widely used to predict the mammary health status of quarters and cows (Barkema et. al., 1999), the suitability of milk for human consumption (Smith et. al., 1999), and monetary losses to producers due to mastitis. Increased cell counts indicate increased inflammation, very likely caused by intramammary infection (Harmon, 1994).

The most important factor affecting the SCC of milk from a quarter, cow or herd is the infection status of the quarter. Various authors have reported average SCC for uninfected quarters to be 170000 to 214000 cells/ml of milk or a geometric mean of 106000 cells/ml. Somatic cell response of infected cow will depend somewhat on the pathogen present. Minor pathogens such as *Corynebacterium bovis* and coagulase-negative *Staphylococcus* averages 227000 cells/ml. Animals infected with major pathogens such as *Streptococcus agalactiae, Staphylococcus aureus*, Environmental *Streptococci* produce average counts greater than 600000 cells/ml of milk from concern animal. Individual somatic cell counts of a cow are the product of the SCC measurement of milk from all four quarters and the level of production of the individual quarters. The number of infected quarters as well as the total milk production becomes important factors in being able to accurately classify a cow as infected by means of SCC. The dilution effect of normal milk can mask infection.

It has been shown by many authors that high individual somatic cell counts (SCC) are positively correlated with clinical mastitis due to persistent infections especially with *Staphylococcus aureus* (Dohoo *et. al.*, 1982). Fewer studies have examined low or very low SCC herds and cows, but there is evidence that the risk of clinical mastitis is increased with low SCC compared to those with higher SCC (Jones, *et al.*, 1984). As the protective immune responses occur in individual mammary glands, more information on the role of SCC at the quarter level is required to increase understanding of local immunity against pathogens. Many experimental studies have shown that high, or even moderate, numbers of somatic cells in milk protect against infection with both major and minor pathogens. The cell numbers may increase either by mechanical stimuli or by the introduction of bacteria.

16. Polymerase Chain Reaction (PCR) in diagnosis of Bovine mastitis

Efficient control of bovine mastitis requires sensitive, rapid and specific diagnostic test to detect and identify the major pathogens/ bacteria that cause heavy losses to the dairy sector through mastitis. Molecular detection of pathogenic microorganisms based on DNA amplification of target pathogen is unique approach for diagnosis of mastitis. PCR is the highly sensitive and rapid technique for the detection of pathogens causing mastitis. Due to limitations/disadvantages of other methods, recent approaches using molecular techniques such as PCR have been developed to identify causative organisms of mastitis. The PCR based mastitis diagnosis test is about 10 fold faster than conventional microbiological methods (Meiri-Bendek et. al., 2002). Multiplex PCR is the modification to conventional PCR which allows simultaneous screening of multiple pathogens that might be causing mastitis (Phuektes *et. al.*, 2001). Multiplex real time assay for simultaneous detection of *Staphylococcus aureus*, *Streptococcus agalactiae, and Streptococcus uberis* directly from milk was developed to evaluate potential use of multiplex real time PCR in the diagnosis of mastitis. Currently PCR assays for the detection of almost all causative agents of mastitis are available but cost effectiveness is the main limitation with requirement of sophisticated laboratory facilities.

17. Enzyme linked Immunosorbent Assay (ELISA) in Bovine mastitis

A direct capture ELISA used to measure increased polymorphonuclear granulocytes (PMNs) antigens also provides an accurate estimate of the cell counts of the milk as low as 100000/ ml of milk. ELISA has excellent potential for the detection of mastitic pathogen. An ELISA of myeloperoxidase is almost as good as capture ELISA using monoclonal antibodies against neutrophil antigens (Gooray, 1994).

18. Cytokine assay

Recently, significant advances in the identification of nucleic acid markers and other novel biomarkers and the development of sensor-based platforms have developed

(Dasilva, *et al.,* 2012). These novel strategies have shown promise in detection of mastitis. Wide ranges of bovine recombinant cytokines are now identified as a new avenue in mastitis diagnosis, therapy and prophylaxis. Assay of cytokines such as interleukin-2 (IL-2) and Interferon gamma (IFN-ã) could provide a swift, reliable and highly sensitive means of diagnosis. Cytokines are the signals that dictate immune responses in normal and infected udders. Hence, subtle changes in the cytokine network of mammary gland help in early detection and further monitoring and effective control of the disease (Peli et al., 2003; Viguier et al., 2009; Mukherjee and Sahu, 2010; Mukherjee, et al., 2010).

Following steps should be followed for prevention and control of mastitis -

- Healthy Clean environment and hygiene in sheds should be maintained
- Cleanliness at the milker's personal side (e.g. hand washing, nail trimming etc.)
- Proper hygiene at the time of milking and after milking
- Hygienic washing and cleaning of udder before and after milking
- Regular pre and post milking teat dipping with antiseptic
- Appropriate management at drying off
- Treatment of infections by Veterinary officer as early as possible

- Proper follow-up of the prevention programme as suggested by the Veterinary officer
- Provide proper nutrition and balanced ration to the pregnant and lactating animals

To conclude, the diagnosis of mastitis is of paramount importance in dairy animals and is quite easy if proper diagnostics approach is practiced by the skilled Veterinarian. Importance of proper diagnosis of mastitis can not be ignored owing to severity of infection and subsequent losses. It is always better to prevent mastitis through the establishment of good husbandry practices, sanitation, and sound milking procedures and culling of chronically infected animals. As it is stated elsewhere, *Prevention is not only better but also cheaper than cure.*

References

Barkema, H.W., Van Der Ploeg, J.D., Schukken, Y.H., Lam, T.J.G.M., Benedictus, G. and Brand, A. (1999). Management style and its association with bulk milk somatic cell count and incidence rate of clinical mastitis. *J. Dairy Sci.* 82:1655-1663.

Christy, R.J. and Thirunavukkarasu, M. (2006). Emerging importance of animal health economics - a note. Tamilnadu J. Veterinary and Animal Sciences 2(3): 113-117.

Dasilva, N.; Díez, P.; Matarraz, S.; González-González, M.; Paradinas, S.; Orfao, A.; Fuentes, M. (2012). Biomarker Discovery by Novel Sensors Based on Nanoproteomics Approaches. Sensors. 12: 2284-2308.

Dhana, M.R. and Sethi, M.S. (1962). Investigations of mastitis in India. ICAR research series No. 35 New Delhi, India.

Dohoo, I.R. and A. H. Meek. (1982). Somatic cell counts in bovine milk. *Can. Vet. J.* 23:119-125.

Dua, K. (2001). Incidence, etiology and estimated economic losses due to mastitis in Punjab and India – An update. *Indian Dairyman*, 53 (10): 41-48.

Gentle, T.A. and Thompson, R.A. (1990). Neutrophil function tests in clinical immunology. International Clinical Immunology, IRL Press, Oxford UK pp. 51-80.

Gooray, R. (1994). *Vet. Microbiol.,* 42; 317.

Griffin, T.K., Dodd, F.H., Neave, F.K., Westgarth, G.R., Kingeill, R.G. and Wilson, C.D. (1977). A method of diagnosing intramammary infections in dairy cows for large experiments. *J. dairy Res.*, 44(1): 25-45.

Harmon, R.J. (1994). Physiology of mastitis and factors affecting somatic cell counts. *J. Dairy Sci.* 77:2103-2112.

Hicks, R.C., Eberhart, R.J. and Sischo, W.M. (1994). Comparison of microbiological culture, an enzyme linked immunosorbent assay and determination of SCC for diagnosing *Staph. aureus* mastitis in dairy cows. *J. Am. Vet. Med. Assoc.,* 204: 255-260.

International Dairy Federation. (1997). Recommendation for presentation of mastitis related data. Bulletin 321/1997. Int. Dairy Fed., Brussels, Belgium.

Jones, G.M., R.E. Pearson, G.A. Clabaugh, and C.W. Heald. (1984). Relationships between somatic cell counts and milk production. J. Dairy Sci. 67:1823.

Lee, C.S., Wooding, F.B.P. and Kemp, P. (1980). Identification, properties and differential counts of cell populations using electron microscopy of dry cow secretion, colostrums and milk from normal cows. *J. Dairy Res.*, 47: 39.

Leslie, K.E., D.A. Barnum, J.C. McTaggart, A. Bishiri, and R. Swackhammer. (1995). Evaluation of a field-based, selective-media bacteriological test system for diagnosis of intramammary infection. Proc. 3rd Int. Mast. Sem., Tel Aviv, Israel, (S2)66-67.

Locatelli, C., Bronzo, V., Sala, V. and Moroni, P. (2010). The importance of an accurate diagnosis to face mastitis and bacterial resistance. *Large Animal Review* 16(1): 3-6.

Meiri- Bendek, I., Lipkin, E., Friedmann, A., Leitner, G., Saran, A., Friedman, S. and Kashi, Y. (2002). A PCR based method for the detection of Streptococcus agalactiae in milk. *J. Dairy Sci..*, 85: 1717-1723.

Mukherjee, R. and Sahu, B.D. (2010). Cytokines for the diagnosis and immunotherapy against bovine mastitis. Indian Journal of Field Veterinarians 5(3): 47-48.

Mukherjee, R., Jadhav, R.K. and De, U.K. (2010). Expression of L selectin molecule on peripheral leukocyte in response to nisin treatment during acute bovine mastitis. Veterinarski Arhiv 80, 355-364.

Peli, A., Scagliarini, A., Britti, D and Boari, A. (2003). Detection of Proinflammatory and

Regulatory Cytokines in Bovine Milk Using RT-PCR. *Veterinary Research Communications,* 27(1): 779-781.

Phuektes, P., Browning, G.F., Flapper, P., Franklin, N.A.D. and Scow, H.F. (2001). Multiplex polymerase chain reaction as a mastitis screening test for *Staphylococcus aureus, Streptococcus agalactiae, Streptococcus dysgalactiae* and Streptococcus uberis in bulk milk samples. *J.Dairy Res.,* 70: 149-155.

Radostits, O.M., Blood, D.C., Gay, C. C. and Hinchcliff, H.E. (2005). Mastitis, In: Veterinary medicine-A text book of the diseases of cattle, sheep, pigs, goats and horses. 9th Edn., WB Saunders Co Ltd., London.

Ranjan, R., Gupta, M.K. and Singh, K.K. (2010). Diagnosis and treatment of bovine mastitis - a holistic approach. *Indian Journal of Veterinary Research* 19 (2): 37-44.

Schalm, O.W. and Noorlander, D.O. (1957). Experiments and observations leading to the development of the California mastitis test. *J. Am. Vet. Med. Assoc.,* 130: 199-204.

Singh, P.J. and Singh, K.B. (1992). A study on economic losses due to mastitis in India. Indian Journal of Dairy Science 47: 265272.

Smith, K.L. and J.S. Hogan. (1999). A world standard for milk somatic cell count: is it justified? *Bull. Int. Dairy Fed.* No. 345, pp. 7- 10.

Varshney, J.P. and Naresh, R. (2005). Evaluation of a homeopathic complex in the clinical management of udder diseases of riverine buffaloes. Homeopathy, 94(2): 81-85.

Viguier, C., Arora, S., Gilmartin, N., Welbeck, K. and O'Kennedy, R. (2009). Mastitis detection: current trends and future perspectives. 27(8): 486-493.

Wu, J., Hu, H., and Cao, L. (2007) Therapeutic Effect of Nisin Z on Subclinical Mastitis in Lactating Cows; Antimicrobial Agents And Chemotherapy, Sept. 2007, p. 3131-3135.

❑❑❑

Chapter 8

Breeding and Its Management in Pigs under Farm Conditions

S.K. MONDAL, B.H.M. PATEL AND S.K. SAHA
Swine Production Farm Livestock Production and Management Section,
Indian Veterinary Research Institute, Izatnagar, Bareilly - 243 122 (U.P.)

Introduction

In India, pig rearing is traditionally very popular amongst the tribal, backward and economically weaker section of the society. Over last three decades, the zero or marginal input situation of this traditional pig farming is gradually changing with a paradigm shift of the society finding the swine production enterprise more profitable and remunerative. The present day swine production is a profitable enterprise in all parts of the world, including India. The initial sporadic imports of improved exotic breeds by the Christian missionaries and subsequent piggery development programmes taken up by the Government were mainly involved with the swine breeding for either the genetic improvement of the indigenous pigs or performance evaluation of the imported breeds. Since 1945, the gradual increase at the annual rate of 4.6% in pig population in India has indicated a steady growth of the swine production enterprise (Das and Bujarbaruah, 2005). The availability of domestic as well as export market for pork makes it more and more attractive. Moreover, the thrust by FAO for research on less-known species and relatively less remunerative agriculture because of gradual shrinking in average land holding due to societal changes and socio-cultural shift towards increasing acceptance of swine production by wider spectrum of the Indian populace have a holistic impact on today's more comprehensive and scientific pig farming.

This, on the other hand, warrants a more integrated and concerted approach to scientific pig farming involving breeding, feeding, housing and health management. This paper is an attempt to some practical breeding related issues relating to Indian farm conditions. The Indian Council of Medical Research (ICMR) has recommended for 34g/d meat consumption, but the availability of meat was 16 g/d in 2000 with the meat production of 4.25 million tonnes (Das and Bujarbaruah, 2005). This demand-supply gap for meat in general and pork in particular, is gradually widening in these days of escalating protein hunger. Therefore, it is high time to streamline the breeding policy, to identify suitable breeds (preferably two or three) and to understand systematic improvement of indigenous pigs. This improvement in the genetic material of indigenous pigs through systematic breeding and subsequent selection is important for a giant stride in improving this sector.

Traits of economic importance in Swine

While planning for a systematic breeding in pigs for their genetic improvement, the traits with economic importance are considered first. The other aspect of this is the prioritization of choosing the traits either singly or in combination. The main handicap in the breeding of swine is that most of the economically important traits have low heritability estimates hindering the selection of the offspring on the basis of the performance of their parents. Some important traits are enumerated below:

Traits	Average heritability
Performance traits	
Litter size at birth	0.11
Litter size at weaning	0.10
Litter weight at weaning	0.19
Daily weight gain	0.32
Feed conversion efficiency	0.36
Carcass traits	
Loin-eye area	0.44

Back fat thickness	0.47
Carcass length	0.50
Per cent ham in carcass	0.48
Per cent lean cuts	0.31

Breeds experienced in India

The imported exotic breeds were initially evaluated for their performance in various Government farms and then the suitable ones were utilized for genetic improvement of the indigenous stock under All India Coordinated Research Project on Pigs. The location specific breed profiles showed that Hampshire was used in northeastern parts, Large and Middle White Yorkshire as well as Landrace were used in northern, central and most parts of southern India while Duroc and Tamworth were used in western and some parts of southern and eastern India, respectively. The exotic inheritance level was restricted to be upto 75%, except for parts of northern and northeastern India, where the level exceeded upto 87.5%. But the general recommendation for genetic improvement of indigenous animal resources in tropics had restricted the level within 75% (FAO, 1997). Few other breeds like Berkshire, Wessex Saddleback and Chester White could not make a mark for their continuance in the breeding programme. The experience of crossbreeding in India has indicated that the heterosis in F_1 crosses can be well harvested rather than clinging on to the higher yield of purebreds.

Selection of breed and breeding stock in Swine

Once the traits to be considered are decided, it is essential that some important points are duly being taken care of for selecting a suitable breed and the proper breeding stock. Some such points are mentioned below:

Breed	Breeding stock
i) Prolificacy	i) Appearance or type
ii) Ability to weight gain	ii) Size of litter
iii) Temperament	iii) Strength and vigour of litter
iv) Carcass quality	iv) Mothering ability
v) Feed conversion efficiency	v) Milking ability
vi) Nicking ability	vi) Pedigree
vii) Disease resistance	vii) Performance or productive ability
viii) Market demand	viii) Prepotency
ix) Availability	ix) Fertility

Systems of breeding

Conventional breeding systems are well in vogue for improvement of swine genetic resources of the country with their intrinsic merits and demerits. However, the relationship of the partners in mating or breeding to produce progeny is more important while planning for outlining a full proof breeding strategy for any farm. The method of **inbreeding** involving mating of related animals, while intended for developing inbred lines, keeping animals purebred and increasing homozygosity, is also confronted with inbreeding depression in respect to certain important economic traits like growth and reproductive efficiency. Crossing inbred lines can lead to recovery of the vigour lost through inbreeding and at the same time keep the animals 'pure-bred'.

The mating of unrelated animals, i.e., **outbreeding**, on the other hand, is extensively used for achieving good results with regard to performance in its three different forms – outcrossing, grading-up and crossbreeding. While **outcrossing** involves mating of unrelated animals of the same breed for multiplying purebred swine, **grading-up** helps improvement of bulk of indigenous nondescript pigs by involving mating of boars of improved breeds with indigenous gilts/sows. **Crossbreeding** involves mating of two different breeds for best exploiting the heterosis or hybrid vigour on those traits whose heritability estimates are low. Crossbreeding is employed for commercial production of hogs more extensively than any other livestock species. Large experience with crossbreds in India has shown them to be superior over the parental performance in many economic traits. The crossbreds have shown heterosis in mothering ability, livability of pigs, rate and efficiency of weight gain as well as in some reproduction parameters. Keeping the performance of the crossbreds in view, the *criss-crossing* and *triple or rotational crossing* have been developed. In criss-crossing, the crossbreds are bred back to the parental purebred breeds alternatively. In triple or rotational crossing, the females born by crossing breed-I with breed-II are mated to male of breed-III. The female progeny born to such mating is crossed to boars of breed-I and the female progeny born in turn to such mating are crossed to boars of breed-II and so on. The crossbreds born will have 4/7 of the inheritance of the breed of their immediate sire, 2/7 from their maternal grandsires' breed and 1/7 from the third breed involved. In both these systems, the heterosis of the offspring and the milk production capacity of the dams (due to larger litters) are exploited.

Planning for Swine breeding

There is a need for planning for breeding in any swine farm before hand to properly exploit the desirable effects of crossbreeding. The shorter generation interval in pigs is an advantage to the breeders due to the quicker evaluation of performance and accordingly the pigs can be selected as per their evaluated performance. An outline for planned breeding to develop 62.5% Landrace crossbreds in a 150-sow farm is being given below as a ready reckoner.

In a breeding farm of crossbred pigs, ideally the male-female should be maintained at a ration of 1:10 to 1:15 for most part of breeding season. However, maintaining 1-2% more breeding boars is always advisable keeping the lower libido, selective mate-choice, breeding injury and occasional non-specific lameness in view. The ideal time for breeding females, in northern India, is during June-July and again during December-January so that the farrowing can occur during October and April, because the most conducive environmental condition prevails. However, in controlled breeding environment, the gilts/ sows can be bred well throughout the year depending on the market demand. One important point to notice here is the body conformation and body size of the breeding partners. Most often breeding boars become over-conditioned due to unrestricted feeding as well as due to the less time available for the sows to restore the body losses, they come across during lactation (especially when large litters are nursed for 42 days). This incompalitibility in size and condition may encourage occasional mate-choice in boars disturbing the scheduled breeding as per the laid down plan. To overcome this difficulty, it is better to select breeding males as well as females from the same batch/ littermates. Restricted feeding of breeding boars may be resorted to until 15 days prior to scheduled breeding time.

Regular exercising may be provided to breeding males throughout the year during morning and evening; this improves sperm quality and ensures optimum male fertility.

Practical guide to develop 62.5% Landrace crossbreds

Time scale	Breed1		Breed2	Total M:F
June, 2011	Landrace (L)	X ↓	Indigenous nondescript (D)	2:20
October, 2011		**L (50) D (50)**		10:50
June, 2012	L	X ↓	L(50) D(50)	2:20
October, 2012		**L(75) D(25)**		10:50
June, 2013	L(75) D(25)	X ↓	L(50) D(50)	5:50
October, 2013		**L(62.5) D(37.5)**		10:50
June, 2014	L(62.5) D(37.5)	X ↓	L(62.5) D(37.5)	5:50
October, 2014		**L(62.5) D(37.5)**		As per provision

Conclusion

The ever-increasing protein hunger in human, specifically in Latin American countries has already made a shift towards the exploitation of relatively less-known livestock species for their meat producing ability. The concerted effort involving judicious breeding programme coupled with the economic and socio-physical climate should be aimed towards the harvesting of heterosis as well as conservation of the indigenous germplasm. Location specific choice of breed, breeding approach for exploiting the desirable characters should be designed such a way that the exotic inheritance be always kept within 75%. The desirable traits of both the indigenous swine gene pool and exotic purebreds should be suitably harnessed while planning for an efficient selection based on performance.

References

Banerjee, G.C. 1991. *A Textbook of Animal* Husbandry, 7th ed., Oxford & IBH Publishing Co. Pvt. Ltd., New Delhi, Calcutta.

Das, A. and Bujarbaruah, K.M. 2005. Pig for meat production. Indian Journal of Animal Sciences, 75: 1448-1452.

FAO. 1997. Recommendations on genetic improvement of livestock in tropics. Food and Agriculture Organization, Rome, Italy.

Prasad, J. 2000. *Goat Sheep & Pig Production and Management,* 2nd ed., Kalyani Publishers, Calcutta, New Delhi.

Sastry, N.S.R., Thomas, C.K. and Singh, R.A. 1983. *Farm Animal Management and Poultry Production,* 5th ed., Vikas Publishing House Pvt. Ltd., New Delhi.

Website of National Bank for Agricultural and Rural Development, browsed on 29.01.12.